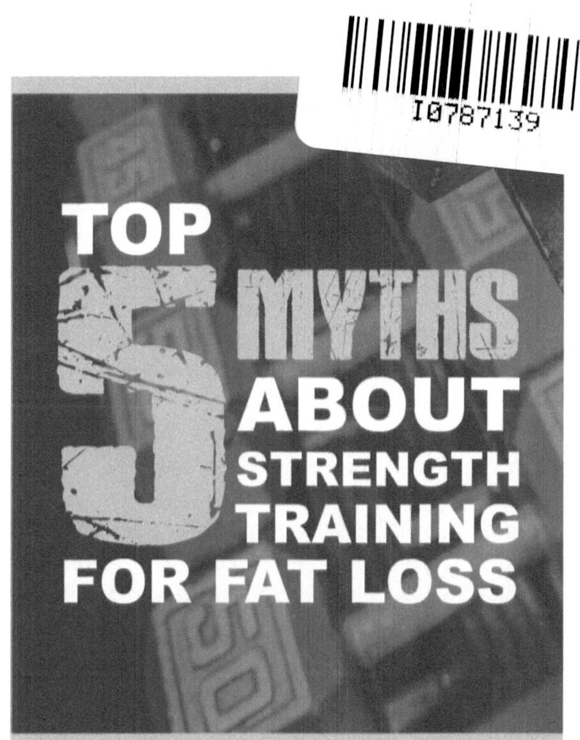
TOP
5 MYTHS
ABOUT
STRENGTH
TRAINING
FOR FAT LOSS

Myth #1: You Can't Skip the Cardio

When it comes to training for fat loss most people turn to running, which happens to be statistically the most common physical activity. It's simple, doesn't require equipment (unless you're a treadmill warrior), and you can do it whenever and wherever you want.
Problem is, it's not the best first-line defense when it comes to fat loss, especially when you also want to build some major strength. Will it halt strength gains altogether? Probably not, but running five days a week and strength-training only two days a week won't get you strong in a hurry.

All exercise burns calories, but not all exercise is created equal. You see, slow, long distance cardio (like jogging) leads to weight loss (notice I said weight loss, not just fat loss). Particularly when long distances are involved, people tend to lose both fat and muscle when running is their primary physical activity. Here's where strength training comes in...

Weight training burns fat AND builds muscle. In fact, a heavy strength training session can burn calories 24-48 hours after the training session. Running will burn more calories than strength training DURING the training session, but running will only burn calories 30-45 minutes post-exercise.

Even more common nowadays is High Intensity Functional Training (HIFT), which is like High Intensity Interval Training (HIIT), only it utilizes a variety a strength training tools -- novelties like kettlebells and ropes, and traditional equipment like barbells and dumbbells.

THE FIT GUIDE: FOR BEGINNERS

A recent study published in *Applied Physiology, Nutrition, and Metabolism* titled <u>Multimodal high-intensity interval training increases muscle function and metabolic performance in females</u>, lasted six weeks and followed two groups who both trained three times a week. Group one did rowing intervals for 60 seconds of work followed by three minutes of rest six times per session. Group two combined the same work and rest periods, but performed three exercises in each 60 second work interval including a strength exercise for four to six repetitions, another exercise for 8-10 repetitions, and a finisher for the remainder of the 60 seconds (something like rope slams). **The researchers found that**: both training strategies led to similar improvements in maximal aerobic capacity and anaerobic power, but the resistance training group showed greater improvements in muscular strength, endurance and athletic performance! The point here is that if you want to burn more calories (by putting on more lean muscle tissue) and make gains in your strength and performance, you are better off performing strength training intervals than you are using a single method like running, biking, or rowing.

Myth #2: Using High Reps & Low Weight is Most Effective

This is probably the most common myth in fitness today, and yet, despite the popularity, we don't have a population full of Spartan warriors. Can higher reps and lower weights be helpful? Yes, to an extent, but when that's ALL you do in your strength training, it can be a problem. If there's no struggle (i.e. heavy weight being lifted), then your body has nothing to adapt to in order to make positive changes. This is why you see that same guy in the YMCA that's been training religiously for 20 years everyday of the week, but he has nothing to show for it, other than staying the exact same size.

You're probably saying, "I know, I know, but I just want to be toned." Here's the funny part folks: Having that "toned" look requires two things -- a decrease in body fat and an increase in muscle size. You actually make it easier on yourself developing that "toned" look when you build muscle while you burn fat.

Using higher reps and lower weights is not designed to build muscle OR burn fat, especially if you never move up to a heavier weight. And when I say "higher reps" I'm talking about anything between 12 and 25 reps, or more! Instead, I recommend a simple principle for progress, and it's called "progressive overload." You gradually increase the weight/resistance used as you gain more strength.

No progress is made with higher reps and lower weight, even if you get tired, so don't exhaust yourself using it thinking you will make the changes you desire to see.

Myth #3: Lifting Heavy Makes You Bulky

Truth – steroids make you bulky. The men and women you see advertising the fancy, expensive supplements you see at GNC; they're most likely not using the supplements they are selling. Instead, they are probably using some form of performance enhancing drug, like steroids. I know this after experimenting with supplements for more than a decade.

I've already talked about the "Firming & Toning" myth using higher reps and lower weights, but getting bulky seems to be the main reason people don't lift heavy weights. Oh, and firming? That just means you have less fat. It has less to do with building strength. If you don't dial in your nutrition and continue to eat poorly while lifting heavy weights, there's a possibility that you will get strong as heck while building muscle, but if you don't lose the fat, you can get a "bulky" look.

Public Perception of Image – look, the whole be as skinny as possible thing went out with the mid-90s. What matters most is NOT what other people look like, or what the public THINKS you should look like. Decide what YOU feel most comfortable with and care less about what people will accept you as. If you need to change how you look to appease people you don't care about, then it's time to make a change. When it all boils down to it, I'd rather be strong and healthfully lean, than super skinny and weak. Get with the times and start loving yourself more, or get new friends. Oh, and a side note, if you're following people on social media that make you feel like you'll never measure up, stop following them. Follow people that inspire and encourage you. Set yourself up for success.

More Muscle Burns More Fat – this is a fact. The more lean tissue that you have on your body, the more calories you burn at rest, doing almost nothing. So why not spend your time trying to put some muscle on as you dial in the nutrition? It will help you burn fat faster.

More Muscle Controls Insulin Better – have you ever considered yourself to be sensitive to carbohydrate-laden meals? Or have you been considered pre-Type II diabetic? Chances are that you may have some form of insulin resistance, or difficulty controlling insulin levels after meals, which unfortunately can lead to increases in fat mass, and a harder time losing fat. Adding more muscle to your body can actually better help control insulin and lead you out of insulin resistance and into insulin sensitivity where your muscles can better absorb and use glucose (what insulin transports) as energy, instead of storing it as fat.

The Athletic Look Is In - We've already discussed how the skinny look is out. So what IS popular? The athletic look. Just look at professional athletes on most team sports. They definitely have some muscle, but they are very lean. Most athletes tend to possess a high amount of relative strength -- that is, pound for pound how strong they are relative to their bodyweight. The more relative strength an athlete has, the quicker and more explosive they can move because they have a lot of strength and very little weight to overcome (their own bodyweight). Again, you choose what's more important to you, because it's no secret that we all want to look good naked.

Myth #4: You Should Train Specific Body Parts

Traditionally, training body parts like chest, biceps, triceps, shoulders, quads, calves, glutes, and core was and still tends to be the most common way of training. That was what I was taught all the way through grade school and into college. But that doesn't mean it's the best way to train for strength or for fat loss. Bodybuilders use BOTH full-body movements and train body parts separately, and they are dang good at it. Chances are, though, you aren't a bodybuilder and you don't plan to compete anytime soon, so lets talk about strength training in a way that gets you the most bang for your buck when it comes to building strength and muscle, and losing fat.

Training with full-body compound movements like deadlifts, squats, push-ups, pull-ups, lunges, and overhead presses will target MORE muscle mass to elicit a bigger response from hormones and metabolism (how your body stores and uses energy/calories).

Reduce Potential for Injury When Training Movements vs. Body Parts – Remember when I told you I used the body-part training method up through my college days? Well, I also started to develop pain and joint issues in my late teens and early twenties because of it. Our bodies were designed to produce movement as a whole unit, all of the muscles and joint systems working together (synergistically, haha), not by themselves in an isolated system. This is why I developed pain symptoms. I was isolating my legs from my hips by doing leg extensions, and isolating my biceps from my shoulder by doing too many bicep curls. Once I transitioned into full-body compound movements, which unfortunately for me was pretty late in the game, I started to see real results in my strength, in my muscle mass, and in my bodyfat and energy. I was taught to avoid "harmful" movements like deadlifts and pull-ups, but as it turns out, those are far better for my body now and for long-term strength.

Everything is attached to everything, and everything works together to an extent – this is how our body works. Even when performing basic tasks like brushing your teeth or standing up from a chair there are multiple joints, muscles, ligaments, and tendons that are working together to produce that movement by the power of your central nervous system (your brain and your spine).

How can we get the BEST response when it comes to strength training for fat loss? Lift more weight (medium to heavy weight) quicker over time (more reps per set, more sets per training session, more volume per training session) all the while using full-body compound movements vesus using body-part focused exercises.

Myth #5: Spot Reduction Works

Here's the truth: you can add muscle to specifically targeted areas of your body, but you cannot lose fat in the same way. Since all of our bodies are different, we all store body-fat in different areas (such as belly, love handles, thighs, hips, upper back, upper arms, neck, etc) and we all lose fat at different rates in different areas. This is based on genetics, gender, physical activity, medications, stress, sleep, diet, and much more. In other words, doing thousands of crunches and other "ab" exercises will NOT target fat loss at your gut. While crunches do target the ab muscles quite well, they won't make your abs visible if they're still covered in a layer of fat.

So, what CAN you do? Focus on lowering body fat by dialing in nutrition, lifting heavy, and upping the intensity of your workouts (by increasing weight, speed of movement, decreasing rest, and recruiting more muscle with full-body movements).

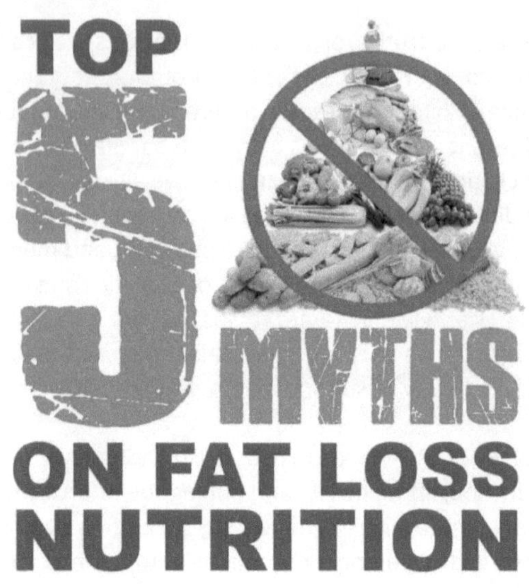

TOP
5
MYTHS
ON FAT LOSS
NUTRITION

Myth #1:
Breakfast is the Most Important Meal of the Day

Truth is, breakfast is your first meal of the day, whether in the morning or afternoon. The word literally means, "breaking your overnight fast," for those of us who don't eat in the middle of the night. If we consider that most Americans habitually eat breakfast first thing in the morning before heading to school or work, then we would also associate breakfast with being the first thing we eat upon waking.   I think where we get lost is assuming that one particular meal, out of any of them, is the most important meal of the day. I will say this, if you are downright ravenously hungry first thing in the morning and it helps you get your day started off right, then eat breakfast, just make sure it's mostly composed of fats and proteins (bacon and eggs anyone?). If you aren't particularly hungry first thing in the morning and you prefer just to drink a black coffee then you may have an advantage when it comes to losing fat. Here's an interesting fact: 90 percent of Americans eat breakfast, and according to the Center for Disease Control and Prevention, close to 35 percent of Americans are overweight or obese. It seems we may not be doing something right.

At the beginning of your day, if you choose not to make food readily available, your body can do some pretty incredible things in the form of using fat as an energy source. Some have even reported having MORE energy in the morning by not eating right away.

When we do put food in our stomach first thing in the morning, we shut down the fat-burning hormones because we don't need to use what we have in storage when we have food in the digestive system readily available for use. It also creates a big eating "window." In other words we are eating food from 7am to 8pm (or whenever you finish dinner), instead of 12pm or 1pm to 8pm. That's 5 or more extra hours of having food readily available in your digestive system. Why is this a big deal?

Mice Study – I know, mice? Just hear me out. There was a study done at the Salk Institute for Biological Studies that had two groups of mice: Group 1 was allowed to eat food whenever they wanted throughout the day with no restrictions; and Group 2 was only allowed to eat food within an 8 hour eating window, beginning in the afternoon and finishing at night. The mice that were given the all-day eating window ended up gaining more fat, developing high cholesterol, high blood glucose, and liver damage. The mice that were given a smaller eating window weighed 28 percent less and had no health problems.

I would like to say that skipping breakfast and extending your overnight fast works for everyone, but it doesn't. Some people just don't jive with it. I say, at least give it a shot for a couple of weeks to see if it makes a difference and make your own decision about it. Intermittent fasting (or extending the overnight fast on occasion) is a great fat burning tool that I use regularly and effectively. In fact, I actually feel hungry less often. But it's not for everyone, especially if you are pregnant or nursing or have major health issues. When in doubt, consult your physician. Just be wary, some physicians are still stuck in the days of the Food Pyramid, so be careful.

So, here's what we talked about: No breakfast = extended overnight fast = fat-burning machine

Myth #2: Carbs are Evil

Carbs are actually a natural energy source for muscles and the brain. It's really funny when we "villainize" carbohydrates like terrorists to our bodies, when some of the healthiest countries in the world with the lowest prevalence of cardiovascular disease and lowest obesity rates, like Italy and Japan, actually consume carbohydrates as a main source of their cultural diet. Oh, and other countries in Africa and South and Central America who thrive off of corn and beans.

The truth is that carbohydrates are helpful when used in the right amounts at the right times. I would also point out that quality of carbohydrates matters as well, as in whole grain vs white-enriched breads, pastas, cereals, and rice. Why? Whole grain, and veggie and fruit sources of carbohydrates are digested slower, contain a higher nutrient content, and provide just enough healthy fiber for our bodies. If you are ACTUALLY gluten sensitive (as I have friends who actually are) then don't eat grains. I'm saying this for the people who have been lied to by the media and gurus who say carbs are evil.

Building muscle and recovering from workouts can be quite difficult without the help of our carbohydrate friends, though I'm not talking about sugary cereals, ice cream, or twinkies.

Fat loss truly all boils down to calories in (what we eat) versus calories out (how we expend energy through workouts and daily activities). Some people are more "sensitive" to carbohydrates and seem to put on weight by just thinking about them, and others can eat them all day without gaining an ounce. Know your body. If you are the first person I mentioned above, then maybe most of your diet should be composed of fats, proteins, and veggies, with some quality carbs here and there. And that's not to say you shouldn't decrease your total calorie intake either. Just don't go overboard with it. Consuming too few calories can actually put your body into a "survival mode" of sorts where it holds on to fat, just in case!

So, when IS the best time to consume carbs when trying to lose fat and gain muscle? The best time to consume carbs is on workout days, and specifically, after the workout. Can you consume them at other times? Yes, but these are the best times and the best days. If your body is limited on the amount of carbs it's given for recovery then it will not only use fat stores to recover from, it will also use muscle tissue, and that's what we don't want.

On non-workout days do your best to stick to proteins, fats, veggies and some fruits that are whole foods loaded with vitamins, minerals, and nutrients that keep you fuller for longer and help you to continue burning fat even when you aren't working out.

Myth #3: Don't Eat After 7pm

This is the one I hear the most. I actually spent time with a potential client who truly believed she couldn't eat after 4pm because it would make her fat! Her mother and grandmother were both competitive ballet dancers, a sport where extra weight is strictly looked down upon, and they were her biggest influencers. For others, celebrities are their biggest influence, and those celebrities tend to swear by not eating after a specific hour at night, as if there's some magic hour after which the horse buggy turns back into a pumpkin.

The truth is, there's no magic time for general food intake. However, eating most of your carbs at night on a workout day can actually be more helpful, depending on how well you digest and tolerate carbs.
In reality, "Your body doesn't store fat more readily during the evening than at any other point during the day." - Alan Aragon, renowned nutritionist

So what does matter? Again, it all comes back to total calories – timing doesn't matter when it comes to food in general.

Lifestyle flexibility anyone? If you're that guy or gal that refused to eat after a certain time, you've probably had friends that eventually abandoned you, or that stopped asking you to go do anything fun because of your food timing restrictions. Give yourself more flexibility and know that there's no "magic" hour after which to stop eating.

Here's what happens when we eat more carbs at night =

We get a more pronounced Growth Hormone release, which means greater muscle growth and for fat-burning.

Greater glycogen storage (i.e. blood sugar that's stored in our muscles) for morning/afternoon training the following day.

Better sleep – Ever eaten a bunch of carbs at night? Puts you right to sleep. Better sleep equals better recovery and better results when it comes to fat loss. <u>These days getting adequate sleep counts more toward fat loss than the amount of food you eat and when you eat it.</u>

Myth #4:
Multiple Meals a Day Stoke the Metabolic Fire

Truth – we burn calories when we eat, it's called the thermic effect of food and it actually contributes to the total amount of calories we expend throughout the day.

Myth – eating more often burns more calories

I was very guilty of eating this way for all of my high school and college years because this is what I was told. This is what was in the magazines and what was widely accepted on the internet by weight loss gurus.

In recent research, both French and Canadian studies found "No evidence of improved weight loss" by consuming all of your calories throughout the day between 6 meals, 3 meals, or 1. When calories are the same (i.e. whether its three 800-calorie meals or six 400-calorie meals dispersed throughout the day) it doesn't matter how many meals you consume. Again, this brings us back to the reigning champion of what really matters: calories/energy in versus calories out/energy expended.

Convenience? Some people love eating 6 meals a day and toting a cooler with Tupperware around with them wherever they go. I don't, and that's why I choose intermittent fasting, and consuming a few meals toward the end of the day, and consuming my largest meal for my last meal of the day. You decide what works for YOU!

Myth #5: You Need to Eat Before You Exercise

Again, this is a big personal preference one. Some people can't move a finger unless they eat something before exercise, and others will feel uncomfortable and end up the victim of projectile vomit during their workout. I prefer to eat after exercise. If you do choose to eat before your workout make sure it's not new food or food that you can't digest easily. It's typical to avoid dairy-based foods before a workout for most people, not because it's bad, but because it tends to cause irritability or indigestion when not given time to digest.

Digestion takes time. Protein digests at a rate of 1g – 10g per hour! So just because you eat 50 grams of protein 30 minutes before your workout doesn't mean your body will actually use it during the workout.

There is some evidence to show that training in a fasted state (no food in your tummy) leads to more muscle and less fat over time.

Hydration (drinking proper amounts of water) and sleep have a bigger impact on your workouts than what and how much you eat before your workout.

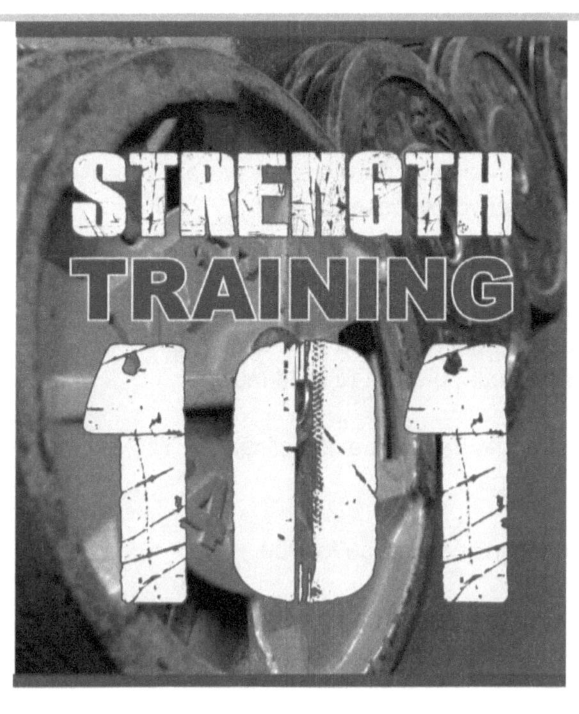

STRENGTH
TRAINING
101

What Is Strength?

Strength, in the most simple terms, is the <u>ability</u> to <u>apply</u> <u>force</u> <u>against</u> <u>resistance</u>.

A resistance could be a barbell, your bodyweight, a machine of some sort, or a large stone. Doesn't really matter what you choose.

Although you CAN build muscle by strength training, strength training and building muscle are not one in the same. For right now, let's stick to strength because it will increase your potential to build muscle.

Can strength training be complicated? Yes, if your career is on the line.

But it doesn't need to be for you.

You want to be as strong as possible to:
    A. Improve your quality of life
    B. Make more money
    C. Be a badass
    D. All of the above

All of these are good reasons.

One of the biggest hang-ups with people when it comes to getting started with strength training is that it seems so complicated!

The truth is it's not. It's actually very simple.

So, why does strength training need to be simple?

Because you don't need the intimidation of complexity to hold you back from getting started.

And because chances are you have a lot on your plate: freinds, family, business, money, bills, vacation, etc.

So let's keep things simple.

Building strength requires 3 simple steps:

1. Do something
2. Be consistent doing that something
3. Make that something more difficult/challenging over time

If you continue following these steps, I guarantee you will get strong, and continue to get strong for a very long time.

Let's break it down:

- **Do something** - well, you can't start getting strong if you NEVER get started. Start with one or two things. Maybe it's push-ups and bodyweight squats. Maybe it's walking up a flight of stairs. Maybe it's curls. Whatever it is, you gotta do something. Got it?
- **Be consistent doing that something** - being consistent means you do it more than once. Not only do you do it more than once, you do it frequently. I recommend starting with 3x/week. Most people find it difficult to see a noticeable change doing something less than 3x/week.
- **Make that something more difficult over time**- here lies the key. Your body is always adapting to whatever stimuli you give it. If you want it to adapt towards increased strength you must give it

something to overcome. Clear on that? This means over time you must do one or some of the following to your exercises:

- Add weight - move more weight than last time
- Add reps - do more reps per set than last time
- Add sets - do more total sets with the same reps
- Decrease rest between sets - rest less between sets of the same number of reps
- Add speed - move the same weight more quickly than previously
- Do more work in less time - same number of sets, reps, and weight used last time, but all done in less time

Next, we discuss the best exercises and the ideal number of sets and reps for building strength.

Best Exercises for Building Strength

There are tens of thousands of exercises and exercise variations out there.

You don't have time for that, and neither do I.

That's why I want you to stick to just 5 movements when getting started, or even if you've been in the iron game for a while.

They're known as the fundamental movement patterns because they are the foundation of all movements we do as humans. Note, I said not the ONLY movements we do as humans, but the foundation. In other words, most movements tend to originate from these.

They are:

1. Push
2. Pull
3. Hinge
4. Squat
5. Lunge

What the what?

Here are some common examples in the same order:

1. Push-up
2. Suspension/TRX Row
3. Kettlebell Deadlift
4. Kettlebell Goblet Squat
5. Split squat

When getting started (or re-started) simply stick to these five exercises.

As you grow in your strength with these exercises you will soon have a foundation that will allow you to move on to more intense and more complex versions of these movements.

Here is an example of what's to come:

1. Barbell Bench Press
2. Weighted Chin-up
3. Barbell Deadlift
4. Barbell Back Squat

5.   Single Leg Squat

Do not stray from these five patterns. Get really good at these and focus on these alone… for now.

Stop making things so complex!

Next, we talk sets and reps.

Sets and Reps for Strength

This is probably THE most common question in the strength training world.

"How many sets and reps do I need to do to build strength?"

Great thing is there are dozens of studies out there on this very subject.

But don't worry I've sifted through all of them.

The biggest conclusion that sums them all up is this:

1 to 15 reps per set produced the greatest results for building strength.

And performing 3 or more sets per exercise produced the best results for building strength.

Can you perform more than 15 reps per set and less than 3 sets and still see gainz?

Yes, but evidence (and my personal experience) shows that the BEST way to build strength is with 3 or more sets of 1 to 15 repetitions per set.

So, we got that out of the way!

Now, what does this mean for you? (with excitement)

I have the perfect blueprint that works for just about anyone.

And, you can use just about any exercise.

Begin with 5 sets of 4 reps.

In other words, find a weight, or resistance, or difficulty that you can perform 4 reps with excellent form.

This means that on a scale of 1 to 10, with 1 being a walk in the park and 10 is extremely difficult, the weight you choose should be a 7 or an 8.

It's quite challenging, but you can also perform multiple sets with the same weight for the same number of repetitions.

So, on Session 1 you did 5 sets of 4.

On Session 2 you are going to do 5 sets of 5.

On Session 3 you are going to do 4 sets of 6.

And on Sessions 4, 5, and 6 you are going to do 4 sets of 8, 3 sets of 10, and 3 sets of 12 respectively, all using the same amount of weight you used to complete those 5 perfect sets of 4 on Day 1.

Simple.

After Session 6 is completed we start all over with 5 sets of 4, only with more weight, more resistance, or more difficulty depending on the exercise you are using.

Use a weight that's, again, a 7 or an 8 on a scale of 1 to 10. This should be more weight than you used for the last 6 training sessions.

Continue these steps until you are as strong as you want to be.

Once you have reached a certain level of strength this concept will no longer apply, but we'll wait till you get there. That will be for a more advanced e-course.

Here it is again to recap:

5 sets of 4
5 sets of 5
4 sets of 6
4 sets of 8
3 sets of 10
3 sets of 12

In the next and final section we will put it all together to get you started toward creating your own strength training program that actually gets you strong!

Putting It All Together

Let's recap.

First, we defined "strength" and really just broke down the idea of getting "stronger."

Now you know that strength is the ability to apply force against a resistance, and getting stronger is training your body to apply more force against a greater resistance over time.

The key is you need to do something, be consistent doing something, and make that something more challenging over time.

Second, we talked about what exercises are best for building strength.

With thousands of movements out there we decided to stick to 5, just 5.

Push, pull, hinge, squat, and lunge.

More specifically, when getting started we stick to push-up, row, kettlebell or dumbbell deadlift, kettlebell or dumbbell goblet squat, and the split squat.

Third, we talked about the ideal number of sets and reps for building strength.

The coolest part is the answer was based off of lots of research and experience.

Begin with 5 sets of 4, then the next session do 5 sets of 5, then 4 sets of 6, 4 sets of 8, 3 sets of 10, and finally 3 sets of 12.

The only thing left to do is get started!

Still not sure where to start?

Once you find a great place to workout, here's how you can get started:

Decide how many days per week you plan to train and set aside that time and block it out.

Blocking it out is a must, otherwise most people tend to just let anything get in the way of their training sessions, but not you!

I recommend finding 3 or more days per week that you can train.

If you train at home all you need is 20-30 minutes max.

If you train at the gym, just be sure to give yourself enough time for travel.

Before each training session make sure you know how many sets and reps you are setting out to do and how much weight you are using. This will make sure no time is wasted.

I highly recommend doing some sort of warm-up even if for 3-5 minutes. A jog around the block or hitting the jump rope will do just fine.

Once you've set your schedule in stone, set aside time, and decided on the exercises to use it's time to get to work.

It's okay to combine two movements back-to-back for the sake of time. This is called a "superset."

Some great examples are:

- Deadlifts and push-ups
- Squats and rows
- Split squats and push-ups or rows

Heck, you can combine three movements back-to-back if you want. It's best to choose 1 push, 1 pull, and 1 lower body exercise for this combo.

An example is push-up, row, and squat.

Whatever you choose, be consistent, use the set and rep plan I provided, don't lift more weight than necessary, and you'll be on your way to a double bodyweight deadlift and repping 20 chin-ups in no time.

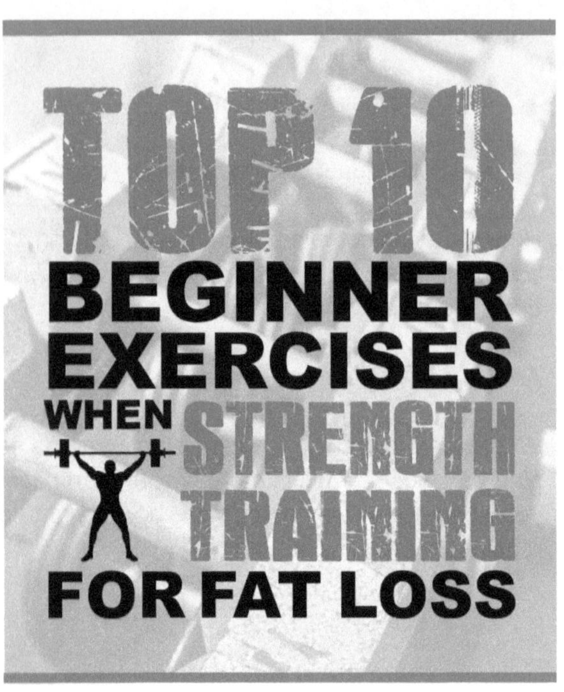

Introduction

One of the biggest roadblocks for people once they make the decision to get back on track with their training, especially when it comes to fat loss, is not knowing what exercises to use. Unfortunately, we have the kind of culture that is counter to simplicity, consistency, and the tried-and-true. Truth is, we don't need the sexiest, flashiest, shiniest new exercises or equipment to get great results.

When I'm training myself or any of my clients I always remind myself to go back to what works:

- Keep it simple
- Keep it consistent
- Progressively add more

When you combine the above principles with the following exercises, you are guaranteed to lose fat while you build muscle. Oh yeah, that's a real thing. You don't have to lose all of your fat before you start strength training, and if you think strength training is going to make you bulky, sluggish, or overweight, please refer back to the Top 5 Myths About Strength Training for Fat Loss.

All of these exercises have some things in common that make them so great for losing fat while building muscle:

- *Full-body.* All of these movements utilize large amounts of muscle mass, which means a better hormonal response and more calories burned.
- *Compound.* All of these movements use multiple joints at the same time like hips, upper back, shoulders, elbows, knees, and wrists, as opposed to isolating a single joint like bicep curls or leg extension in a machine.
- *Ground-Based.* Simply put, all of these movements require you to stabilize yourself under your own power as you perform the movement, whether you are on the ground or suspended on a pull-up bar. The opposite involves sitting on or in an exercise machine, and allowing that machine to fit your body into specific angles and ranges of motion, which can limit how well your body moves and how many muscles and joints you can utilize for the exercise. Plus, ground-based movements are closer to real life. Outside of sitting in a car, there aren't too many situations in your day-to-day life that involve you doing something where you aren't based on the ground.
- *Allow for Heavy Weight to be Lifted.* Remember, lifting heavy weights puts the body in prime mode to build

muscle and burn fat, so why not choose exercises that allow you to lift as much weight as possible? Doing contralateral single-leg deadlifts on a BOSU ball with your eyes closed doesn't allow you to lift heavy weight. And you better believe lifting your own weight with pull-ups, pushups, handstands, and rows involves lifting heavy weight, especially if you have a lot of weight to lose. Bodyweight movements, such as these, also tend to be favored mostly because of the other five bullets in this list.

- *Functional.* Push, pull, squat, lunge, hinge, rotate: these are functional movements that we use daily. So why not make them the foundation of your strength training program?

- *Requires Minimal Equipment.* We're all on a budget, right? So why choose exercises that require expensive specialty tools? Feel free to use dumbbells, kettlebells, barbells, weight plates, resistance bands, bodyweight, sandbags, punching bags, large stones, heavy books, cinder blocks, car tires, car rims, chains, other car parts, or heck, use the entire car for "sled" pushes. Get creative, and don't limit yourself to conventional tools.

#1: Push-Ups

Hands down one of the most fundamental and underrated strength movements, even though the push-up is an upper body focused exercise, I would promote it as a full-body exercise. If you are doing it correctly, you'll be engaging the glutes, abs, upper back, calves, shoulders, triceps, and more! You'd be amazed how many so-called "fit" people cannot perform a single quality pushup. I'm talking no sagging or high hips, elbows not bowed out, forearms vertical, upper arms brushing the sides of the torso throughout the movement, and going all the way to the floor. I require everyone I train to master the pushup before they have a shot at a bench press or floor press. Learn to master your bodyweight first. The push-up is one of those timeless exercises that you should always have as part of your program, whether once a week or everyday. If you are unable to do one on the floor, the best way to progress to the floor is to use an elevated surface. We setup a barbell at a specific height using the j-hooks to accomplish this. I rarely recommend the knee pushup as it places the torso, hips, shoulders, and elbows at a disadvantage. If you don't have access to a power rack you can use a sturdy table, desk, bench, or chair, or the back of a car or truck! Lastly, you should not be "feeling" the pushup in your shoulders or elbows; instead, you should place the work on the triceps and upper back. Check my YouTube channel for a tutorial.

#2: Overhead Push Press, Handstands & Handstand Push-Ups

This is another one of those upper body movements that must engage the entire body; otherwise the movement is unstable and lacks its full strength-building potential. Very few people realize that in order to press the weight overhead, you need to transfer force from the ground through your body to the hands. The bar itself is producing a downward force that you must overcome, aka gravity. IF you have weak legs, glutes, torso, or upper back you will have a difficult time stabilizing your arms and transferring force from the ground. I threw handstands and handstand push-ups in there for a few reasons: 1) If you don't have a barbell, kettlebell, or dumbbell to press overhead this is a great alternative to develop overhead pushing strength. 2) It's a great movement to learn altogether as you will develop upper body strength and control you just can't get from pressing an object overhead. In other words, you will work muscles you never knew you had, especially because of the balance factor, which can help you break through plateaus in the overhead press. 3) Sometimes we just need to have a little variety to keep things fun. I've spent entire sessions just practicing freestanding handstands, hand-walking, one hand holds, cartwheels, and round-offs. Talk about developing some extreme athleticism.

#3: Pull-Ups & Chin-Ups

The king of all upper body pulling movements, you can do lat pulldowns for the rest of your life, or you can move up to the true measure of strength. I have nothing against lat pulldowns, but sooner or later you need to graduate. If you can't do pull-ups yet, then the next exercise I talk about below will help get you there. You can also use a partner or some heavy-duty resistance bands, like we do at our gym. When building strength in the pull-up you have a few variations at your disposal: 1) Both palms facing forward. 2) Both palms facing you. 3) One palm facing you, and one facing away. 4) Using a neutral grip where your palms face each other. Unfortunately, this variation can only be used if you have access to a neutral grip bar. There are some after-market add-ons you can sometimes fit to standard pull-up bars. Whichever version you choose, keep those hands shoulder-width apart. Don't go crazy with a super wide grip. As you pull up, avoid flaring the elbows out to the side, and don't make your shoulders do all the work. Instead, engage your upper back by depressing your shoulder blades and activating your lats (those large wing-like muscles under your armpits that run along the back side of your ribs). And make sure you use a full range of motion, i.e. always start with the arms fully extended and pull up until the chin is completely over the bar.

#4: Rows

The row is not a common exercise most people think of when it comes to building a solid foundation for strength, mostly because it's not considered one of the traditional "sexy" exercises. If you are just starting out, or trying to rebuild strength lost long ago then don't skip the rows! Here are 7 solid reasons you need this in your strength-training program: 1) Easy to learn; 2) Improves posture in a functional pattern; 3) Increases grip strength; 4) Teaches people to use their "other core" (aka your glutes); 5) Increases pushing strength, as in your push-ups; 6) First step toward the pull-up. If you can't do one yet, this is an incredibly effective way to work your way up to it, literally, haha; and 7) Requires minimal equipment or space. All you need is a pair of rings, a TRX, or simply use a barbell setup on some J-hooks in your power rack. You can also row a barbell, kettlebell, or dumbbell from a modified wide-stanced lunge position. Just make sure you keep your hips low and your back flat.

#5: Squats

Some will argue that this is THE king of ALL exercises, but I would argue that it is not, but don't let that downgrade its ability to add some incredible strength and size to the legs and glutes. If you hold the weight in front of you as in a barbell front squat or a kettlebell goblet squat you will also build a rock solid torso because you can't hold all that weight out in front of you without being strong in your mid-section. When you are squatting please remember that EVERYONE will squat differently, some with a narrow stance and some with a wide stance, some with feet pointed straight ahead and others with feet pointed out. Find what works best for your body. There is NO standard that you have to fit. Just make sure you don't experience pain while doing them, whether that pain is in your hips, knees, or ankles. Also, on the contrary to what many people will tell you, squats don't destroy your knees, that is, as long as they are done correctly. That's why it is so important to find a squat position that works best for your body. As long as your heels don't leave the ground, your shoulders don't fall forward, your back doesn't round, and your knees don't cave in you should be just fine. Try to shoot for at least getting low enough so that the upper legs are parallel to the ground. If you can go down until the hamstrings touch the calves, then even better. Again, it all boils down to how your body is shaped, from your hips to the length of your femurs, to how your femurs fit inside your hips, to where your bodyweight is distributed, and how much mobility you have in your ankles. Can't squat safely from the start? Try using a high box to squat down to, then work your way down to a low box, and eventually no box. I've had success using the box with many clients.

#6: Deadlifts

Okay, here it is, the undefeated champion of full-body strength movements! The only other exercise that could compete is not actually a single exercise, but two: the clean and press. But we are here to talk about the deadlift. Why is the deadlift considered the best full-body exercise and the squat isn't? Most of it has to do with the incorporation of the upper and lower back, shoulders, forearms, and hands, and the fact that it starts from a dead position, as opposed to the squat where the person can lower themselves and use a "bounce" to spring out of the bottom, which is fine as it uses the body's natural elasticity found in ligaments, tendons, and muscle tissue, but it's easier to do anything with a bounce versus having zero momentum. The problem is, deadlifts have gotten a bad rap over the decades for causing low back injuries. There is some truth to this, but it's only when deadlifts are performed with horrible form OR when too much weight is used. How do you stay safe? Find a form that best fits your body, like with the squat, and stick to it, in addition to only performing max efforts on occasion instead of every other training session. If that weight moves only a couple of inches in the first 3 whole seconds it's too much weight. Don't feel comfortable using a barbell? Kettlebells are a great substitute, as are single-leg deadlifts if you have them down. Trap bars, those metal hex-shaped bars, are also a great tool as they center the weight with your body, instead of pulling the weight from in front of you. Don't feel comfortable deadlifting from a conventional stance (feet hip width and arms just outside your legs)? Try using a sumo deadlift, modified sumo deadlift, or a Jefferson deadlift. All are great options. Last key thing about deadlift: you will get more out of this exercise if you lift heavy weight and stay in the 3-6 rep range per set. Notice, even if you stay in that rep range, but you lift weight that's considered a 5 or less on a scale of 1-10 (10 being extremely heavy) then you won't reap the benefits of this exercise because your body isn't being challenged.

#7: Lunges

Can't forget the single-leg work (also known as "unilateral" work). Lunges and their variations are great for hitting those muscles that don't get used during their two-leg cousins, the deadlift and squat. I've used lunges with my clients and with myself to help increase my squat and deadlift numbers. There are many "stabilizer" muscles that keep your knee in place during a lunge that you can't target with the squat or deadlift. Additionally, the lunge can sometimes help people work in a greater range of motion than they could hit in the bottom of the squat, and you can sometimes get an active stretch on the trail-leg hip, further increasing your future performance of the squat. Stick to reverse lunges and walking lunges most of the time, but you can try forward lunges and split squats (where your feet don't move, only your hips move up and down as your knees and hips bend and extend).

#8: Farmer Carries

One of the simplest exercises you could ever perform. Notice I said simple, not easy. This exercise involves holding heavy weights in each hand and carrying them for a long distance or an extended period of time while maintaining a solid and flat upright posture. This exercise is also a form of a "loaded carry," which means you can feel free to hold different sized weights on each side, carry one overhead and one at your side, or hold both at chest level. What's unique about the farmer carry is it's carryover into the deadlift with it's emphasis on developing the back and shoulders while forming a strong grip. The thicker the handles, the heavier the weight, and the longer the objects are held the more you will get out of it. When holding kettlebells or dumbbells do your best to keep the weights off of your hips and legs, otherwise you're cheating the exercise. Don't forget you have to lift the weight off the ground first, so train the lift off the ground like you would the deadlift: keep the back flat, shoulders above the hips, and hips above the knees. Keep the shoulder blades back as you walk and whatever you do, don't let your shoulders crumble and roll forward. Work on carrying more and more weight over time, and everything else you do in the gym will just get easier.

#9: Sled Drags & Pushes

Even though sled drags and sled pushes require a specific piece of equipment, you can make one for free or very little money or just put your car in neutral in an open parking lot or driveway and you are set! Pushes and drags are such a great tool because, like the farmer carry, they are easy to learn and simple to perform. You almost can't screw the movement up. Sleds will also develop your entire body, especially your glutes, hamstrings, quads, upper back, shoulders, and grip! When pulling the sled forward or backward, keep the shoulder blades back and maintain a tall chest while keeping the straps in line with your torso. When pushing the sled keep your hips in line with your hands, forming a straight line from hand to hip along your elbows, shoulders, and back; this will allow you to push with as much force as possible.

#10: Sprints

I'm not talking about a jog, or a fast jog, or a run, or a fast run. I'm talking about an all out sprint like your life depends on it! One of the most primal movements you can do, and when not performed lazily, it can elicit some powerful hormonal and nervous system responses that are downright animalistic. Keep the sprint distance short as in 10-40yds or go for time and keep it in the 10-20sec time frame per set. Even though the sprint is a basic movement, it's not so easy to learn, especially if you haven't done them for a while or if you have tight hips or poor posture. Here are some things to keep in check: Keep arms at 90 degrees at the elbow with hands open; move your hands from cheek to hip with every swing; avoid moving your arm across your body, and instead move your arms straight forward and backward; emphasize the back swing NOT the forward swing since the harder and faster you push back into the ground behind you the harder and faster the ground will propel you forward; keep your head in line with your spine and don't lean back; strike the ground on the ball of the foot or the mid foot; avoid taking long strides as they can literally put the "brakes" on. Lastly, when you decelerate at the end of the sprint, slow yourself down by gradually lowering your hips until you are in a modified lunge position, and avoid leaning back and overstriding at all costs as you might end up with a pulled hamstring or hyperextended low back.

#11: Bonus – Hip Thrusts/Glute Bridges

I put this as the "afterthought" #11 because these two exercises are very unconventional and "go against the grain" when it comes to tradition. However, once you get past the tiny discomfort and unfamiliarity that accompany these exercises you will soon see how powerful they are at developing the glutes, while adding strength to the hamstrings and low back on the side. I've personally used both the glute bridge and the hip thrust for the past few years and seen a big carryover to my deadlift, squat, sprint and jump performance, and an increase in glute and hamstring size. The best way I know how to perform these is with a barbell and a really thick barbell pad that some people use for back squats. I purchased one on Amazon made by Hampton for about $35 and it works great. When performing the glute bridge, your shoulders and feet will be on the ground. When performing the hip thrust your shoulders will be elevated (on something like a flat weight bench; I use an empty beer keg) and your feet will be flat on the ground. Make sure that the bar and pad are centered over your hips and that you stabilize the bar by extending your arms and pressing the bar firmly into your upper legs. Take in a deep powerful belly breath and drive through the heels as you explosively squeeze your glutes to elevate the hips. Make sure that you completely lock out your hips at the top of the movement before lowering the bar back to the floor. If you are unable to start using 45lb plates on each side, which is common, it would be helpful to have bumper plates the are 10lb, 15lb, or 25lb since they elevate the bar high enough to get the legs under.

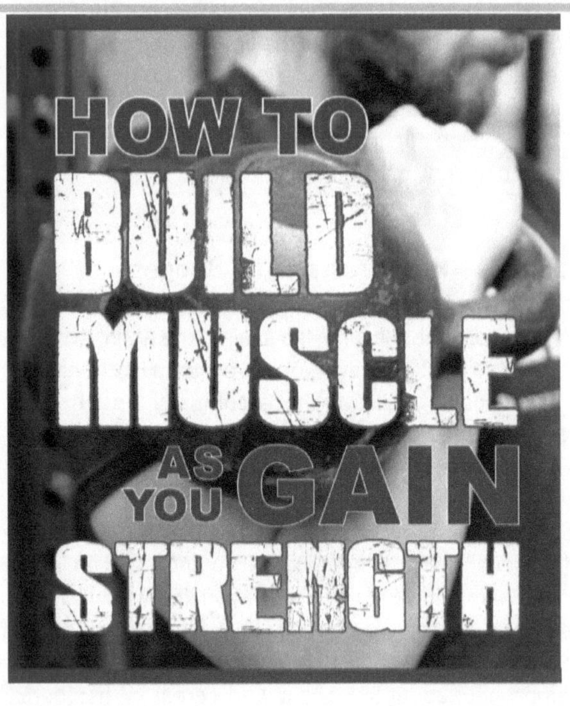

HOW TO
BUILD
MUSCLE
AS YOU GAIN
STRENGTH

So you want to get strong and lose some fat if possible, but dare you also venture out to build some muscle?

It's okay, everybody wants to. The problem is no one's willing to admit it; even those people who claim they just want to be "firm" and "toned."

Why would anyone want to put on extra muscle?

The real reason is why WOULDN'T they want to put on muscle?

Well, for most people they don't want to transform into some ginormous iron-eating meathead with so much muscle they can't safely drive a passenger car.

Lucky for you, it requires eating dumptruck loads of food and a little "juice" if ya know what I mean.

If you really do want that firmed and toned look, you're going to need to put on some muscle. There's no way around it. Though I have met people who literally want to train without gaining an ounce of muscle. Once I pick up my jaw off the floor I kindly say goodbye to them and wish them luck.

My point is it's perfectly normal to want to put on some muscle, and unless you plan to step on stage in Vegas, there's a really good chance you won't gain too much muscle.

Now that you have confirmation that it's okay to build muscle, what's the point, other than looking better?

Well, the biggest reason is that over time more muscle means you eventually develop a higher potential for building strength.

When you first begin strength training a lot of your initial strength gains will be due to your nervous system learning movements, improving control, and getting better at creating and maintaining tension throughout your muscle system.

Your body will also become more effective at utilizing energy, and you may see some gains in muscle. But you want more so you can get stronger, right?

Let's get started.

Here's are some of the questions you can expect answers for as you read this eBook:

- Is it possible to gain muscle and lose fat at the same time?
- How long will it take to put on a significant amount of muscle?
- How much muscle can I expect to gain?
- What kinds of food should I be eating?
- What foods should I avoid?
- Can I still build muscle if I don't eat meat?
- How much do I really need to eat to put on more muscle?
- How often should I eat?
- Can I have cheat meals?

- What else can I do outside of training and nutrition to optimize my strength program?
- What are the best practices for building muscle?

---

1. Just how much muscle can you gain? Is it possible to build muscle and lose fat at the same time? How long will it take?

The short answer is: It depends, yes, and it depends.

The amount of muscle you put on is dependent on some things that are out of your control like gender and genetics, and on some things within your control like stress, sleep, food, and training style.

The Rock is a great example of a genetic freak (in a good way). He's massively muscley, but he's also hella lean. Unfortunately, not everyone has these genetics. Let's look at the different types of genetic giftings.

In terms of genetics there are three basic types of people when it comes to putting on muscle:

- I Type - these are the men and women with a more slender build (narrow shoulders and hips) who can eat Cheetos and Big Macs all day and hardly gain an ounce; they also tend to have a hard time putting on muscle - not that they can't, they just really have to work at it.

- V Type - these are the men and women who are naturally athletic and have broader shoulders with a moderate to narrow waist and powerfully lean hips. They can build muscle and lose fat fairly easily by changing their diet and training program.
- O Type - these are the men and women who have a naturally broad or thick build and tend to put on mass pretty easy, sometimes even by just thinking of food. Strength comes fairly easily to these people, but getting lean might be a challenge - again, not impossible, just tough.

Of course there are hybrids of these three types, just know that genetics play a big role in how much muscle you can build.

And let's not forget gender.

Ladies, adding muscle to your upper body is possible, but it won't come as easily as it does for men who just naturally have more testosterone and more upper body mass. You DO tend to add muscle to your upper legs and hips fairly easily. This is why ladies be lovin' deadlifts and squats.

Men, you are almost the exact opposite. Though there are some genetically gifted studs out there with natural tree-trunk legs, most men will tend to either gain moderate amounts of muscle easily in both upper and lower body, or moderate amounts of muscle in the upper body and not so much in the lower body.

Either way, have grace for your gender and genetics people. They're out of your control anyway, remember?

So what about those things within your control when trying to build muscle?

When it comes to building muscle there are many factors you can directly affect for your benefit: sleep, stress levels, proper food intake, and how you train.

If all of this is optimized, which rarely ever happens for the non-sponsored 9-to-5er, here's what you can expect for gaining muscle:

- **Excellent progress** - expect to gain 1-2 lbs of muscle every 2 to 4 weeks.
- **Average progress** - expect to gain about 1lb of muscle every 4 weeks.
- **Slow progress** - expect to gain less than 1lb of muscle every 4 weeks.

So, if you want to gain 10lbs of muscle at an average pace you can expect to do so in about 40 weeks, or 10 months. 1 year is probably a more reasonable mark.

Most people prefer this process to be a little quicker. Just make sure that if you plan to try and pack on muscle quicker while also planning to lose fat, it's probably not a good idea to stuff yourself all the time by going on a "see food" diet.

Yes, you can build muscle and lose fat at the same time, but the process is much more gradual and takes much more patience. Contrary to popular belief it is not necessary to gain a bunch of fat in order to gain muscle - this comes from people who tell themselves this so they can eat whatever they want and because they lack patience.

Let's take a look at optimizing the things you can control.

---

2. What Kind of Foods Should I Be Eating/Avoiding? How Much Food and How Often Should I Eat? What if I Don't Eat Meat?

This is a small list of some very loaded questions, and to be honest there is far more to discuss here than we can put in this eBook, but there are some basic principles that will help you get started.

If you are looking for some more in-depth nutrition help, whether it's for improving performance in the gym, putting on some muscle, or making some major progress in your fat loss, we have a Certified Sport and Exercise Nutrition Coach available for our members.

The type of foods you eat will depend on your goals (in this case we're focused on building muscle), genetics, and gender.

For example, carbohydrates can really help an I-Type and a V-Type person pack on some muscle as it aids in workout recovery and can help in shuttling protein to the muscles that need it most. However, for our O-type friends, even though they will benefit from keeping carbs in their diet in low to moderate amounts, it's best if they stick to getting most of their calories from proteins and fats.

In the end, all three types of people will benefit from adding more protein to their diets. And if you are looking to build muscle there's a good chance you will need to

take in more calories during the week than you currently
are if you want your body to see a change.

Let's keep things simple.

The following is a breakdown of how many calories per
pound of bodyweight you might take in if your goal is to put
on muscle based on your activity levels:

- Sedentary (minimal exercise) - 14-18 calories/lb of
  bodyweight
- Moderately active (3-4x/week) - 16-20 calories/lb
  of bodyweight
- Very active (5-7x/week) - 18-22 calories/lb of
  bodyweight

If you are trying to lose fat while you build muscle it would
be wise to stick to the lower end of these caloric
recommendations.

Now, what about macronutrients. Maca what?

Macronutrients are the three nutrients the body requires in
large amounts. They are:
- Proteins
- Fats
- Carbs

The amount of each you take in will largely depend on
your body type. Your body is an indication of how well, or
not well, your body utilizes each type of nutrient.

Here's a breakdown of what percent of your total daily
calorie intake should be proteins, fats, and carbs based on
body type:

- **I-Type**: Protein - 25% | Carbs - 55% | Fats - 20%
- **V-Type**: Protein - 30% | Carbs - 40% | Fats - 30%
- **O-Type**: Protein - 35% | Carbs - 25% | Fats - 40%

So, if you're an I-Type who weighs 120lbs who is moderately active and you're looking to gain muscle you should be taking in between 1,920 and 2,400 calories (16 to 20 calories/lb of bodyweight) per day. Your macronutrient breakdown might look like this if you chose to go with 1,920 calories per day:

- **Protein**: **120 grams of protein** (0.25 x1920 calories = 480 calories → 480 calories / 4 calories per gram of protein = 120 grams of protein)
- **Carbs**: **264 grams of carbs** (0.55 x1920 calories = 1,056 calories → 1,056 calories / 4 calories per gram of carbs = 264 grams of carbs)
- **Fats: 43 grams of fat** (0.20 x1920 calories = 384 calories → 384 calories / 9 calories per gram of protein = 43 grams of fat)

Is there some wiggle room in this? Absolutely.

Find what works for you and your body and your schedule and budget.

Here are some good examples of foods in each category:

Protein
- Lean red meat/beef
- Salmon
- Eggs
- Boneless skinless chicken
- Ground turkey
- Plain Greek yogurt

- Whey or plant protein supplements without artificial sweeteners

Vegetables and Fruits (with each meal)
- Broccoli
- Cabbage
- Cauliflower
- Spinach
- Mixed berries
- Tomatoes
- Oranges

Other Carbohydrates
- Black or Pinto or Red Beans
- Whole oats
- Whole wheat bread
- Rice (white or brown, white can be better for gaining muscle, and brown for losing fat)
- Lentils
- Potatoes
- Yams

Good Fats
- Raw, unsalted mixed nuts
- Avocados
- Extra virgin olive oil
- Coconut oil
- Fish oil
- Flax seeds

Drinks
- Water - at least half your bodyweight in ounces; double that if you workout

Just remember this is not an exhaustive list. There are many more foods that could be considered "good."

The source of the food can have an impact as well on your muscle gain, especially when it comes to protein. Grass-fed beef, wild-caught salmon, free-range eggs and chickens, etc. This level of quality isn't necessary, but it's a good idea if it fits your budget.

Fruits and vegetables should be a staple no matter what since they provide another type of nutrient: micronutrients - which we need in much smaller quantities than macronutrients above.

How often should you eat?

Frankly, it really doesn't matter as long as:
- You are getting in the total number of calories you desire each day
- You are recovering from your workouts
- You would consider your energy levels good most of the time
- You're not feeling deprived or overfull
- You're seeing the results you want to

What this boils down to is this…

If you prefer to eat breakfast, lunch, and dinner, then do that.

If you prefer to skip a morning meal and just eat in the afternoon and evening, then do that.

If you're a huge fan of 6-8 meals a day and it doesn't stress you out packing and prepping all of those meals, then do that.

What matters most is that you are seeing evidence of the outcomes you want to see: speedy recovery from workouts, high energy, feeling satisfied, and seeing the results you're going for.

If not, then you need to change things up!

For our friends who choose to avoid meats, it is very possible for you to put on muscle too.

Here are some key things to keep in mind:

- Most meatless sources of protein also have a lot of carbs which will add up quickly to daily calories
- Unlike meat sources, meatless sources of protein like beans, rice, and lentils are not complete proteins. A complete protein provides every essential amino acid - proteins our bodies cannot make, but must get from outside sources. Therefore, when not eating meat, it's a good idea to combine protein sources like beans and rice at a meal to make sure you are getting a "complete" protein.
- When seeking meatless protein sources, including protein powders, it's a good idea to avoid soy.

The last thing I'm going to talk about in this section is something everyone wants to know about - cheat meals.

What's a cheat meal?

It's that meal that's always on your mind, even when you're eating right.

It's the meal you're talking about when you say, "You know what? If I didn't have to be so disciplined all the time I'd love to "go to town" on a _________ filled with _________ and topped with __________, that I'd down with a cold __________."

Maybe it's a double-decker cheese pizza stuffed with peanut butter and jelly deep fried and covered in sugar. I don't know, use your imagination.

Truth is, the longer you withhold from having food you enjoy, the more likely you are to go a little overboard when you do.

Most cheat meals are loaded with large amounts of the infamous carbohydrate, usually in the form of bread, pasta, cereal, waffles, pancakes, and many forms of sugar.

Why carbs? Because they seem to be the thing people think are evil and will ruin your progress.

Funny thing is those same people have demonized carbs to the point of depriving themselves enough of them that their performance and body composition has gotten worse.

If you want to put on muscle, carbs are going to be necessary. Believe me it took a while for me to realize this because I was strict Paleo for so long. When I reintroduced carbs I was able to lift more, put on more muscle, and actually got leaner!

Back to cheat meals...

Are they okay?

Absolutely.

In fact, having a cheat day can actually be beneficial given the rest of the week you've been extremely ON POINT with your nutrition - meaning you never slipped up, and you actually kept your daily calories a little lower than normal by a few hundred calories.

When's the best time to have a cheat meal/day?

Soon after a solid training session in the gym, preferably a heavy lifting day - deadlifts and squats work great for this. There's no magical secret exercise to do before a cheat meal. Just make sure you train like you mean it.

After a hard workout your body is craving nutrients to be used for recovery - mostly protein and carbs. You're more likely to use the carbs right after a training session, rather than storing them as excess fat, especially since you were at a caloric and carbohydrate deficit the rest of the week. A cheat meal/day also let's your body know that you're not dieting yourself away. Your body has a built in survival mechanism (a mix of glands and hormones) that will literally slow down your metabolism to the point where building muscle and losing fat will nearly come to a halt.

Just don't use cheat meals/days multiple times a week as an excuse to get huge and not go into "survival mode."

So, with food out of the way let's talk about training.

3. Training to Build Muscle

Training for strength and training to build muscle are not always one in the same. There's definitely some crossover, but there are specific principles that apply to training to build muscle that don't necessarily apply when building strength. Let's take a look at some of those principles.

Much of what people know about building muscle comes from what they hear from passersby at the gym or from their favorite jacked celebrity or from their muscle and fitness magazine.

Building muscle is still a science that is being studied and tested regularly. Funny thing is much of what we know and apply today was learned from Arnold's day when he was training in the original Gold's Gym and would spend hours in the woods squatting heavy things and eating steaks and drinking wine. Okay, that last one is a rumor, but I believe it to be true.

 So let's begin on what we do know about building muscle through reliable research and studies, and for this I turn to a Strength and Conditioning Research review that I subscribe to. This review is authored by a biomechanics researcher, Chris Beardsley and, a strength and conditioning coach and front-runner in sports performance research, Bret Contreras.

After sifting through dozens of muscle-building studies from the last 30-40 years they came to a few conclusions about developing muscle mass:

- Training programs should focus on increasing volume - or doing more overall sets and reps (either in individual workouts or by training more often).
- Use full ranges of motion - each rep goes all the way up and all the way down.
- Train to muscular failure when possible - during times of slow recovery don't train to muscular failure.
- Use exercises that involve both an eccentric and concentric component (up and down) - versus just a down component or just an up component.

As you can see, most of these principles already apply to strength training - more volume, full ranges of motion, and using eccentric and concentric components.

When training for strength going to muscular failure may not be the best idea. Is it wrong? Not really, but doing it often with heavy strength training movements can lead to injury and slow down your strength gains.

Now that we have the sciency researched stuff out of the way, what are the "secrets" to building muscle?

Well, depending on who you talk to you're going to get a lot of different answers. In the end, you will need to experiment with a little bit of everything and find out for yourself.

Here are some principles that I've found to be extremely helpful when building muscle. Some of these may go against what research shows us, and some agree with the research:

Use specific rep ranges for specific muscles - some muscles are built with muscle fiber types that are designed for endurance (higher reps) and some are designed for explosive power (lower reps). Therefore, train specific muscle groups with specific rep ranges to elicit growth. Here are some examples:

- Biceps - 10-15 reps per set
- Triceps - 6-10 reps per set
- Upper Back - 6-10 reps per set
- Shoulders - 6-10 or 15-20 reps per set
- Glutes - 15-25 reps per set
- Quads - 15-25 reps per set
- Hamstrings - 6-10 reps per set
- Calves - 15-20 reps per set

Again, this is not an exhaustive or exact list, but it can be extremely helpful when setting off to train specific muscle groups.

Notice how all of these rep ranges are focused on specific muscles, versus being focused on movements or movement patterns like we do with strength training.

With strength training we are developing strength using movements like squats, deadlifts, and presses. With muscle-building we are developing muscle in specific areas that are best trained in isolation.

If building strength is your priority then I recommend doing your strength training work first, and then finishing your workout with some isolation work for putting on some muscle. After all, when building muscle it's not about how much weight you lift.

When building muscle, not only do we recommend targeting specific muscles with specific rep ranges, we also recommend combining those rep ranges with other key principles:

- Time under tension - slow down your reps.
    - It's actually helpful to slow down the eccentric (or lowering) portion of the lift. During the eccentric portion your muscle fibers are lengthening, but they are also having to produce force - this creates a lot of stress.
    - Typically with strength training, the eccentric portion, though controlled, is much more passive and is just what we have to do to get to another concentric rep. Try lowering the weight for 3-6 seconds. Don't spend any time at the bottom or top of the lift, and make the concentric component about 1 second. The exact seconds don't matter, just slow down your reps.
- Shorten the range of motion - I know the research recommends using full ranges of motion, but sometimes a full range of motion can give your muscles too much of a break at the top or bottom of the lift, like in a bicep curl.
    - Remember, we're trying to increase time under tension and taking breaks shortens that time under tension.
    - Use shorter ranges of motion at your discretion.
- Mind to muscle connection - when you train a muscle, focus on it with your mind.
    - Seriously, rather than just squeezing out curls to get to the end of the set try putting

your focus on the biceps muscles being worked.
  - Some research has shown signs of increased muscle growth by focusing on the muscles being worked.
  - This is definitely one of those principles used by the old school bodybuilders that hasn't been fully proven yet.
- 60 second rest periods - this isn't an exact science, but we need to rest long enough to recover before the next set, but we also don't want to lose the "pump" we've created from the last set.
  - Somewhere between 60 and 120 seconds seems to be the jam. Find what works for you.

Take these principles as you will. The best thing you can do is try them out for yourself.

Just remember that no matter how many "secrets" we use to build muscle, how much you build and how fast you do it ultimately depends on the limiting factors we discussed earlier: genetic potential, gender, and hormones.

Now that we got all the cool training stuff out of the way let's take a look at some of the other factors that significantly affect muscle-building progress.

---

4. What else can I do outside of training and nutrition to optimize my muscle- building, strength-gaining program?

Don't worry, this isn't a huge list.

We're mainly just talking about two things: stress and recovery.

Stress is an interesting one. We all could use some major relief from stress in our crazy lives, but we also need to create stress in the gym to build some muscle.

Here's the deal, too much stress can cause some major problems. In fact, excessive stress can keep you from building muscle at all.

Whether it's family, your job, money, social media, the internet, poor food choices, or school, it's nearly impossible to rid yourself completely of all these stresses. Therefore, instead of quitting our lives to build muscle, it's probably a better idea to manage our stresses with our gym time, while optimizing recovery.

What's recovery? It's the time when you actually build muscle! It's the time outside of the gym when your muscles relax, absorb nutrients, expel waste products, and rebuild.

The three most important components of recovery are:

1. Food
2. Water
3. Sleep

Pretty simple, right? Notice there are no magical supplements in this list, or even massage.

These three simple components give you the most bang-for-your-buck when it comes to recovering fully and properly.

We already discussed food and water. Make sure you're taking in enough of both. If you're not recovering from your workouts you might need more food. If you pee yellow all the time, then you definitely need more water.

If food and water are both in check, but you're still not recovering, then sleep is most likely the culprit.

Most people need 8-10 hours of sleep, yet most people get 4-6 hours of sleep. I get it, we gotta work, but we also need to binge watch Netflix. But remember, Netflix won't help you build more muscle.

It is crazy how much recovery goes on in our sleep - hormones, nervous system activity, nutrient transport. There is so much that happens in our sleep that our body cannot do, or has a hard time doing, when we're awake. Sleep is like the magic elixir, but no one is doing it!

We suggest following a few simple principles to get more sleep:

- Create a routine - go to sleep at the same time each night. Your body needs rhythm.
- Avoid caffeine consumption later in the day - some people shouldn't consume caffeine past noon, and others do fine quitting by 4pm.
- Make sure your belly is full - ever try going to sleep while you're hungry? Doesn't work. Carbs are great for putting you to sleep. :)
- Dim the lights about 45-60 minutes before going to sleep - the low light will prep your brain for slowing down and relaxing.
- Make sure your room is dark and cool - blackout shades and fans are great for this.

There are many more things that can help you get better sleep, but we're not doctors so this will be a good start for you.

Just know that even with your training and food intake on point, building muscle will be challenging if you are overstressed and not recovering from your training.

If you're still not sure where to start, or you could use some help getting pointed in the right direction come check us out at Snohomish County Strength. We have all the equipment you need, along with a staff of experienced coaches who are there just for you. Snohomish County Strength is all about building muscle, increasing strength, and putting in the work.

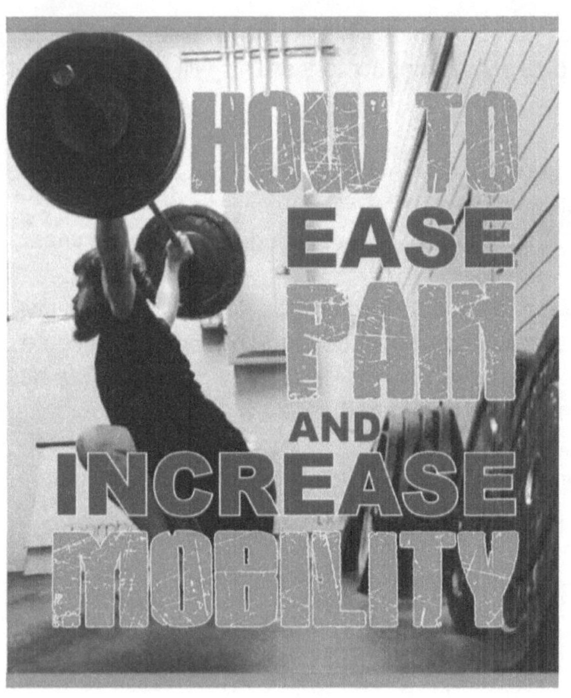

Disclaimer: This book was not written by a medical doctor, nor is it intended to replace anything your medical professional has prescribed for you. All of the information below was gathered from experience with hundreds of clients and athletes of all ages, genders, and abilities, and should only be performed AT YOUR OWN RISK. Jon Chacon is dissolved of all medical responsibility of the reader.

1. Optimal Breathing

It's funny, when most people think of moving better and getting out of pain the LAST thing they think of is to work on improving their breathing!

How we breathe determines how we move. From the day we are born we all naturally breathe using our diaphragm (pronounced die-uh-FRAM). Don't worry, it's not a special breathing tool that only the "privileged" kids got to use. It's actually inside of you, and it's this dome-shaped muscle that spreads across the lower portion of your ribcage. The diaphragm is there to help us breathe.

We all know that our lungs are up in the top portion of our ribcage, but the muscles and tissues in and around the ribs are NOT built for breathing, at least, they're not designed to do all the work. Stupid ribs, they don't even do anything - except provide critical protection for our heart, lungs, and major veins and arteries.

Here's where the diaphragm comes in. Like I said before, the diaphragm is a muscle, just like your heart is a muscle. Fortunately for us, the heart pumps without us having to think about it – or we'd die. The diaphragm, on the other hand, isn't one of those "set-and-forget" muscles that just does its job without needing to be told.

During most of our childhood we instinctively breathe the right way using our diaphragm – meaning we use our diaphragm muscle to create a vacuum that helps our lungs take in oxygen and exhale CO2. As we got older, our posture got worse and we got more stressed. As a result, we stopped using our diaphragm and started relying on our chest and neck muscles to breathe.

Breathing this way causes two big problems:

1) It causes us to build and hold tension in our chest, neck, shoulders, and upper back. Over time this causes our shoulders to round forward and our neck and upper back to develop pain.
2) It causes us to not be able to take in an optimal amount of life-giving oxygen for our brain and muscles, and to exhale all of the carbon dioxide (waste product) that we produce. In the end, we end up not getting enough of what we need, and we hold on to some of what we don't need.

Bottom line: getting out of pain begins with getting your breathing right. In other words, retrain your brain to use your diaphragm to do the heavy lifting for your breathing. Using your diaphragm will remove the stress and tension from your chest, neck, and shoulders and will give you more energy since you can take in more oxygen and exhale all the CO2 you produce.

Here's how to get started with diaphragmatic breathing:

- Lie on a comfortable flat surface on your back with your knees bent, feet flat on the floor and hip width apart, and back of your head resting on the ground.
- Place one hand flat on your belly (where your diaphragm and abs are), and one hand on your chest (where your lungs and ribcage are).
- Next, we're going to focus on learning how to "belly breathe" using your diaphragm instead of your chest.
- Begin by taking in a nice deep breath inhaling through your nose only - your focus should be on ensuring your

- belly is rising more quickly and fully than your chest; if it's not, then make it happen.
- During the inhale you should take in as much air as possible until you cannot take in anymore. When I say "nice deep breath," I mean it!
- Next, begin to exhale out of your mouth as slowly as possible - your belly should be caving in as your diaphragm is working to push air out of your lungs.
- At first, you will work on inhaling for 3-5 slow seconds, pausing for 3-5 slow seconds, and then exhaling for 3-5 seconds.
- Do this breathing exercise for 10-20 breaths per day (absolutely do more if you have time - all we're trying to do is re-teach you how to use your diaphragm), so the more you do it the better.
- Eventually, you want to make it a goal to inhale for 20-30 seconds and exhale for 20-30 seconds - at this point you really learn to "control" your breathing through the use of your diaphragm. When you reach this level, not only are all the right muscles working, but you become extremely efficient at using air to the point where nothing is wasted. The pause between inhale and exhale is not a big deal. If you keep it in the 3-5 second range you should be good - we don't want anybody dying.

Over time you will also notice muscles in your torso getting stronger - your abs, your lower back, and even the pelvic floor muscles (below all your guts).

Using your diaphragm not only helps you to breathe better, it's also an effective replacement for a weightlifting belt. You know - those super thick leather belts you can win in professional wrestling matches? No wait, not those. I'm talking about the weight belts people wear in the gym to aid in bracing and protecting their spine and torsos during heavy lifts.

Beyond just providing protection, a weightlifting belt is very effective at forming a strong link between lower body and upper body. This allows the lifter to effectively transfer forces from the ground to the hands and upper back. Think of a deadlift or a back squat - LOTS of force going through the torso.

So, how do we use our diaphragm to form a brace?

This is done by using your diaphragm to take in a deep breath that you hold while simultaneously squeezing all of your ab muscles (along with a bunch of other muscles surrounding your torso, but let's not make this complicated). This will help you lift more weight, and safely. More weight safely lifted = stronger.

2. Neutral Posture

If diaphragmatic breathing was a superhero and part of a dynamic duo, the second member of the duo would be neutral posture. The two work hand-in-hand, and dare I say *synergistically*. They can both work independently from each other, but they provide the best results when they work together!

Neutral - sounds boring right? It may be boring, but it's going to help you move more weight and stay out of pain. Sound good?

When I talk about neutral posture I'm referring to your spine, that's it.
Check it out, neutral posture is the sweet spot between two extremes - hyper flexed (spine bent forward) and

hyperextended (spine bent backward). Most people tend to spend a lot of time in the first one - slouchy, shoulders rounded forward, neck sticking out.

Not only does this forward position cause injury when lifting heavy things, it's also a terribly ineffective way to produce force. In other words, force transfers very well in a straight line (neutral posture), and not so well in a bent or rounded line (forward posture). Think about doing an overhead press. To lift as much weight as possible we want the force to transfer from the floor up through your hands overhead in a straight line

Whenever we lift heavy weight the force we generate first goes down into the floor, which in turn comes back up through us (Newton's Third Law - look it up). In order for us to lift optimally (i.e. without leaking energy), it's a good idea to not be in any kind of bent position, whether forward or backward.

Neutral posture is also the best way to give our hips and shoulders a large range of motion to operate in (range of motion is how well a joint can move unobstructed). When we are in a bent-forward posture our shoulders have a hard time moving to the overhead position because our shoulder blades are pulled apart, and our glutes can't work in a squat or a deadlift because the hips aren't allowed to move freely. All you need to know is bent-forward = bad, and neutral posture = good.

How do you get into neutral posture? Simple, just remember to keep the following three points in line at all times:
1. Back of your head
2. Space between your shoulder blades
3. Back of your tailbone (pretty much where your belt might sit)

You can hold a PVC pipe, broom stick, foam roller, or any other kind of light-weight straight object along your spine to see what it feels like to line up these three areas. Just know this doesn't work if you only have two out of the three areas in line - all three need to be in line. If they are not and you cannot get into the right position comfortably, then you may need to work on gradually getting your head, neck, shoulder blades, and hips back into a neutral position.

This is something you can do as you work on your breathing, and it can be done just about anywhere. Remember, if neutral posture doesn't feel natural right now there's a good chance you've formed your current posture over the course of a few years, maybe even decades. Just know that's it's going to be a long term process that won't happen overnight. Have some grace for yourself.

We can work on our posture by:

1. Constantly being aware of, and adjusting our posture throughout the day (for most people this means pulling the shoulders and head back - you may need to adjust your computer screen or the driver's seat in your car to make a major impact).
2. Breathing diaphragmatically instead of in your chest.
3. Combining massage and stretching on a regular basis to your trouble areas (more on this later).

3. Soft Tissue + Stretching

Ever had a massage? If not, I'm sorry. If so, you know what I'm talking about. When you get a massage (good massage) you should feel relaxed afterward. The reason you went to get one in the first place is that you had so much "tension" throughout your body, probably in your back, neck, shoulders, arms, or even legs.

Here's the deal, even if you train/lift weights regularly and you never go to failure you are bound to create excessive amounts of tension over time to the point of feeling stiff. (Notice I said excessive, which is more than normal. We all need tension in our muscles for our bodies to work properly.)

Eventually, you stop moving as well as you used to, and you might even start to feel pain in some of your joints where you didn't have pain previously. It might end up in your shoulders, back, hips, knees, ankles, elbows, wrists, you name it.

The odd thing is unless you sustained a serious injury directly to that joint, there's a good chance that the pain in the joint doesn't stem from the joint itself. Rather, it stems from having excessive tension in the muscles and tissues above and/or below the joint. For example, elbow pain may be coming from excessive tension in the forearms, or in the triceps since both muscle groups have an attachment to the elbow joint.

When you get a massage you feel relief because tension is released. We hold our tension in a tissue that surrounds all of our muscles, joints, ligaments, and tendons. It's called Soft Tissue (or Fascia in the medical world (pronounced fă-SHUH)). This is why you hear people say, "Did you do you soft tissue work?" All they are asking about is if you did some self-

massage to get rid of excessive tension in your trouble spots.
We can develop excessive tension from the following:

- Working out
- Sleeping the wrong way
- Sitting at a desk in front of a computer all day
- Performing a repetitive movement over a long period of time
- Being mentally stressed out
- And many more

Overall, you can't avoid excessive tension, and it's not always going to accumulate in the same places.

How does massage work?

When we accumulate excessive tension it presents in the form of "knots" in our soft tissue. Basically, our soft tissue gets waded up like a rat's nest - all the tissue is criss-crossed and out of line. In order to get it back in line we need to apply pressure to get it to move, and believe me it can be stubborn. There's a good chance that when you hit the right spot it's going to be a little uncomfortable...okay, it's going to be A LOT uncomfortable. We just don't want it to be painful. If you ever experience any numbness, tingling, or burning sensations stop immediately. When that happens something isn't right.

You're going to continue applying slow, deliberate pressure to your tense areas until that soft tissue flattens out and eventually realigns as it once was. When you do it right you should feel great relief in your joints and your overall movement quality should improve tremendously since you won't have anymore obstructions.

There are many tools that you can use in the gym and at home to do your soft tissue work. In the gym, you've probably seen foam rollers - these are great for doing soft tissue work. At home, I've used baseballs, softballs, lacrosse balls, and even a sturdy Nalgene water bottle. Whatever you use just make sure that it works for you and that it is structurally sound and won't collapse under pressure.

The arena of soft tissue work and self-massage is huge in the fitness world, and there's just too much to go over in this eBook. Just stick to these principles when doing it:

- Apply pressure to the muscles and tissues surrounding joints, NOT on the joints or directly to bone
- The pressure you apply should be slow and deliberate, not fast and hasty.
- Do it everyday - hitting soft tissue work is much less effective when only done once or twice a week. Taking just 3-5 minutes a day can make a HUGE difference.
- Always do your soft tissue work in a good position - we just talked about neutral posture and diaphragmatic breathing, adhere to both when doing your soft tissue work. It's not a good idea to contort yourself in stressful positions as you try to relieve tension.

Oh, I almost forgot to talk to you about stretching. The good thing is soft tissue work, breathing, and posture are extremely important and will make your stretching more effective.

Let's illustrate how soft tissue work goes hand-in-hand with stretching.

Let's say you like to chew gum, but you only chew it for a couple of minutes. And when you are done chewing the gum you stick it in the freezer for later. I know, weird right? Stick with me (haha, get it?). Later in the day you crave that piece of gum you were chewing earlier so you grab it out of the freezer, only now it's hard and stiff. You throw it in your mouth and start chewing. Eventually it starts to warm-up and it becomes more flexible.

When you go in for your workout your tissue tends to be like that frozen piece of ABC gum. Before you start stretching that frozen tissue it's a good idea to "chew" it up a little bit to make it more pliable, and more open to being stretched. This is why stretching is so much more effective AFTER soft tissue work. Can you stretch without doing soft tissue work? Absolutely, but it will be more effective if you do both.

What kind of stretches you ask? There are far too many to list, but I would recommend one or two for these major areas: Ankles, Hips, Upper back, Chest.

You can stretch more areas, but these four will give you the most bang-for-your-buck if you are short on time. Two great resources for stretching that put out a lot of great free content are Dr. Kelly Starrett of Mobility WOD and Jill Miller of Yoga Tuneup. I have subscribed to Dr. Starrett's Premium Mobility WOD membership and it's totally worth the $9/month.

Soft tissue and stretching can be performed before and/or after your training, or it can be done before going to bed or in the middle of the day. Just make sure it works for you!

4. Stop Working Through Pain

Alright, let's start wrapping things up here. What I want to
finish with is how to deal with pain.
Pain is one of the most discouraging things in the gym,
especially when you have been consistently putting in the work
to get strong, put on muscle, and lose some fat.
The conventional wisdom behind "no pain, no gain" would tell
us to simply push through the pain and suck it up! But in this
case, conventional wisdom is an idiot.
Pain is simply a negative signal from our brain. It's a built-in
protective mechanism that prevents us from using the area
affected. So it's not actually your shoulder that hurts, it's your
brain telling you there is something wrong with that area. It
could be strained, hyperextended, torn, or inflamed. Either
way, your brain is smart and it's telling you to stop using the
affected area.
Are there times to work through pain? Definitely. These are
typically in emergency situations. If you are working out at your
home or in the gym you're most likely not in an emergency
situation, unless your pride got the best of you and you put too
much weight on the bar for a bench press and you are getting
crushed under the weight.
My point is, most situations allow us to back off and not
aggravate the pained area. When we continue to push through
pain our bodies naturally compensate to pick-up the slack of
the pained area. For example, let's say your shoulder hurts. As
you continue to train, your upper and lower back, elbow, and
wrist on that side are going to have to pick-up the slack by
doing jobs they weren't built to do. Since they are taking on
more than the usual work they will eventually accumulate pain

and start to affect more areas of the body that extend far above and below the originally affected joint!

The best thing you can do is swallow your pride and find something else to do that does not cause the pain to surface. Allow your body to do its job and heal. If your shoulder hurts, there are thousands of exercises you can do using the rest of your body. In fact, studies have shown that continuing to train other parts of the body that are not in pain will speed up the recovery of the parts that are in pain. Continuing to train allows your blood to carry waste products out and shuttle recovery products into all joints since blood travels everywhere! If you just have to train the affected area, which I know many people will still try to do, then I recommend trying a few of the following:

1. Change the tool - if you typically use a barbell, try using dumbbells, kettlebells, bands, or bodyweight.
2. Restrict the range-of-motion - instead of pressing the weight all the way overhead, try only pressing it to the point right before you start to feel pain. If you're squatting and your knee hurts, you can squat to a box that stops your descent to the point right before your knee hurts.
3. Lighten up the weight
4. Slow down the movement
5. Change the angle - if bench pressing and overhead pressing hurts, try an incline press using an angle right between the two. If regular deadlifts hurt, try a sumo deadlift position.

There's always a way to continue training when suffering pain. It's just not the best idea to work/push through it.

The best things you can do to alleviate pain are:
- Sleep
- Drink plenty of water
- Eat a well-balanced nutrient-dense diet
- Hit soft tissue work regularly
- Continue training everything else

Once the pain is gone, take your time working that joint back into your training and try not to hurt it again - learn from your mistakes!

Pain is almost completely unavoidable when training. It's going to creep in at some point, even with the most perfectly planned and executed program. Just know you're not alone and it's not the end of the world.

Begin with learning to breathe again using your diaphragm and shifting your body back into a neutral posture that's comfortable and so easy to get into it's almost instinctual.

With the breathing and posture down, make soft tissue work and stretching a regular part of your training, and please do your best NOT to push through pain.

Let's do this!

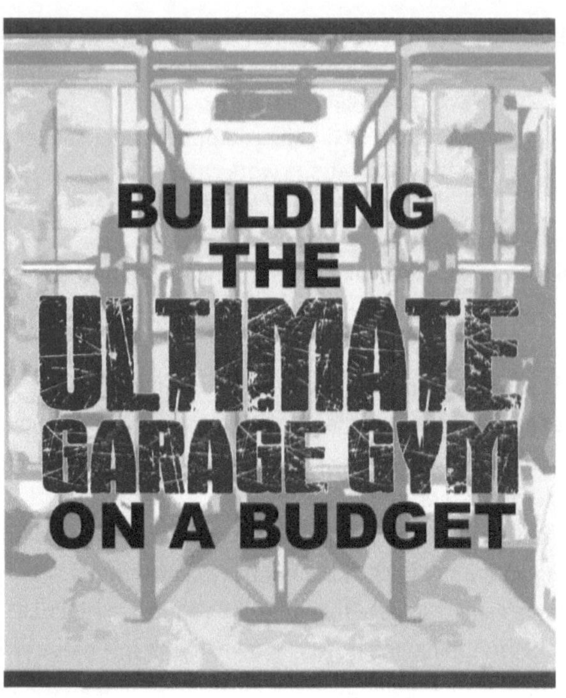

By far two of the most common excuses for not beginning a strength-training program are:

1. *No Money.* Most people don't want to invest in a long-term gym membership or a personal trainer.
2. *No Time.* Most people claim they don't have the time, or the last thing they want to do after just waking up or after a long day is get in the car and travel across town to the local gym.

The best way to get rid of both excuses and set yourself up for success to is to build your own gym. Here are some benefits to building your own garage gym:

- Train whenever you want
- Listen to your own music
- Feel free to use chalk and drop weights
- Cast iron lasts forever and won't break
- No monthly payments
- No weirdos bothering you while you workout
- Buy used equipment using your own budget

Look at it as an investment. Most people who don't succeed have an "expense" mindset where they spend money that's lost forever and so they never spend it because it's a liability. Instead, develop an "investing" mindset. Invest in your health, in your future, in your family, and in your success. Building your own gym is an investment for life. You get to design it how you want it.

Here are a couple of things to consider when deciding on a location:

- *Height.* If you are going to be pressing a barbell with some plates on it overhead, you better have more than 8-foot ceilings. A lot of garages, even ones with finished ceilings, have heights that are more than 8 feet. If the ceiling isn't finished then you're in luck. If the space you plan to use has 8 feet of height or less, then either don't plan to do overhead work, or do it in a seated position. If you plan to do any jump training, a low ceiling will also cause some problems.
- *Walls & Floors.* If you plan on installing anything, like a power rack or a pull-up bar, then it needs to be anchored. The power rack would need to be anchored to the floor (concrete is best), and the pull-up bar will need to be mounted to wooden studs either in the walls or in the ceiling. If the room you plan to use does not have concrete floors you will need to get creative with how to anchor it. I've used

heavy sandbags, heavy dumbbells, or a partner. Some companies manufacture power racks that have built in plate pins the will hold half a dozen 45lb plates. I also don't recommend carpeted floors as they have too much give and can be uncomfortable. I've used them by placing horse stall mats on top of them.

- *Windows.* Decide if you like to have fresh air (if you can't open the garage door), or if you like to see outside. A window can also be a problem if it's in the wrong spot and if your workouts get a little out of control, so just be mindful of it when choosing.
- *Space.* The absolute smallest square footage I've used is about 24sqft, no bigger than a 4'x6' horse stall mat. Hopefully, that's not what you are working with. The best minimum square footage when working with a barbell is 48sqft, or two side-by-side horse stall mats. Remember, you will also need to move equipment in and out of the area.
- *Noise.* Avoid choosing a space where you can't crank your favorite tunes or drop weights without bothering everyone else around you. If you are in an apartment you might want to either stick to kettlebells, dumbbells, and bodyweight exercises, or hopefully you live on the ground floor. If you own a house, make sure your training sessions won't disturb family members who are sleeping, doing homework, reading, or trying to carry on a conversation.
- *Temperature.* Decide how much you care about temperature regulation. If you don't mind putting on a bunch of layers and wearing fingerless gloves in the winter, and if you are okay with using fans that cool your naturally-occurring sweat in the summer, then you won't have too much to worry about. If, however, you know that your motivation to train will be seriously lacking if your garage/room is too hot or too cold, then make sure you have a plan This could mean investing in a large floor fan for the summer, or getting a space heater for the winter. Just make sure

you have access to outlets and that nothing in the room will cause problems, like using a space heater next to something that could catch fire.

Equipment

Essentials. What you will need at a minimum; this will depend on space, budget, and what you actually want to do. If you are very limited on space and budget then bodyweight training might be your best bet. If you have a decent amount of space and a good budget to work with then you have more options.

- Power Rack – This is a great tool to have because it serves multiple functions, especially if you plan to make barbell lifts a staple. If all you want to do is deadlift with your barbell then you don't need a power rack. Racks are made by various manufacturers and come in different sizes. For the most part, it resembles what looks like a cage with four upright posts that are connected along the ground and from the tops of the post with cross members. Ideally, look for one that has a pull-up bar built right in. The power rack should be made of some thick (at least ¼"), heavy duty metal. Ensure rust is very minimal and that nothing is rusted through or corroded. Welds should be smooth and not rough or sharp (check corners and angles for these). There should be multiple pin holes for the J-hooks (these hold the barbell up). Don't get too crazy with how many holes there needs to be. Ensure all the nuts and bolts are in place. Lastly, make sure it fits your space.
- Barbell – There are A LOT of used barbells out there and most of them are low quality and made in China. A great way to know immediately is how the sleeves (ends of the barbell that actually rotate) are attached. The sleeve end will either expose a hex head bolt (poor quality) or a barely visible snap ring (sign of better or good quality). Physically check the "spin" of

the sleeves. If they barely rotate 1 full rotation with a good spin from your hand then it's probably seen better days. If it spins 1-3 full rotations then you have a pretty decent bar. Also make sure you don't hear any rattling, scratching, or clunking as the sleeve spins. Next, check the knurling (rough part) of the bar itself. Grab it, grip it, and get a feel for it. Does it fit in your hands well? Does it feel too bulky? Does it slip out of your hands too easily? Make sure you like the feel of it. Another indication of a poor quality bar is how thick it is. A standard barbell diameter for a 45lb bar is 28mm. If the bar feels too thick, there's a possibility it's a poor quality bar since manufacturers will save money on cheaper metal, and in order to make the bar strong enough to hold weight they have to make it thicker. Lastly, check for any rust and make sure the bar isn't bowing or bending. If the bar had too much weight on it in the past or was allowed to bounce or drop too often, it could have a permanent bow in it which won't make your training much fun. If there's a little rust, you can take care of it with some gun CLP (cleaner, lubricant, protectant) oil. If there's a ton of rust, just don't buy it – it's seen better days.

- Plates – Look for cast iron plates with a 2" center hole, also known as Olympic style plates. A good starting setup would be the following: 6x45lbs, 2x25lbs, 2x10lbs, 2x5lbs, 2x2.5lbs. Don't get more until you can use more. Make it a goal to use all of them at once eventually. Don't worry too much about rust. Just use some gun CLP oil or some CLR (calcium lime rust) remover. Plates last forever no matter how much rust they have.

- Horse Stall Mats – If you plan to drop any kind of weight and you don't want to cause damage to your floor or your equipment, I recommend investing in some heavy-duty rubber mats. The best kind to get are at least ¾" thick and are usually 4ft x 6ft. They are the same mats they put in horse barns and trailers, thus the name. They are designed to withstand impact from a 1000lb+ animal. You can get them at farm and ranch co-ops or at places like Tractor Supply Co. I've bought many from gyms going out of business or from people who bought too many and needed to get rid of them quickly since they take up space and weigh 80-100lbs each. Try not to buy these new if you can.

- Kettlebells or Dumbbells – I almost put these down as optional items, but in case you either don't have room to use a barbell, don't feel comfortable with a barbell, or just prefer something other than a barbell, then kettlebells and dumbbells are a good choice. The only potential problem is that eventually you will need different sizes to adapt to your increases in strength. This is why a barbell is so versatile because you can have a variety of weight amounts to choose from using different combinations of plates. Now, if I were to choose between getting a couple kettlebells or a few pairs of dumbbells I would choose a couple of kettlebells (one medium weight and one heavier weight, like a 16kg/35lb and a 24kg/53lb for men). Here's why. A kettlebell is capable of being used for far more movements, particularly strength movements like presses, deadlifts, rows, and squats, AND conditioning movements like snatches, swings, and cleans. With dumbbells you can attempt some conditioning movements, but it can be quite tricky. The other great thing about kettlebells is they require smooth dynamic movement, as opposed to abrupt jerky type movement. If you just feel more comfortable with dumbbells, since they are a more well-known conventional tool, then I'd recommend investing in at least 3 pairs that are 10-20lbs away from each other, such as 30s, 40s, and 60s.

- Weight Bench – I put this as optional. Unless you plan to do a lot of bench pressing, you won't need it for much of what I recommend as far as exercises go. Besides, if you have a good power rack, you can perform floor presses, which is basically a bench press except you lay on the floor instead of a bench. If you want a good solid weight bench they can be upwards of $300-$500. I have been lucky enough to find one like this for $75, so it's not impossible. Just know it's a choice and not a must-have.

- Pull-Up Bar – If you opted out of the power rack, you are still going to want a sturdy bar for working on pull-ups or hanging a suspension system from. You can build one yourself with 1-1/4" metal piping, or you can buy a manufactured bar built to attach to wall or ceiling studs. I do not recommend using one of those cheap indoor doorway pull-up bars. They can be useful if you are really in a money pinch, but eventually something goes wrong. You can also just go to the local park to use one for free!

- Rings or TRX – These are great to have around when developing pull-up and push-up strength. In fact, I recommend this as one of the best strength training beginner exercises. Outside of rows, I don't use them for much else. You can now find brand new rings with straps for as low as $35. If you decide to go the TRX suspension system route because of the more ergonomic handle, then I don't recommend buying the TRX. Go with the Jungle Gym made by Lifeline USA. It does the exact same thing for about 1/3 the price.

- Slam Ball or Ropes – These are great tools for conditioning, but you need to have some space available for the ropes, and have a place where you can make some noise. They can also be quite expensive. A 10lb slam ball can be as much as $55 and a 30ft rope can be up to $200!

- Push/Pull Sleds – These are great tools, but they can get expensive, especially the push-type sleds. I recommend building your own pull sled from a $20 tow strap, a few feet of chain, and a large used truck tire. That's how I used to do it. Don't pay any money for the used truck tire, you can ask your local tire shop to point you in the direction of all the old tires they took off of cars.

Where to Buy & How Much to Spend

o Craigslist and garage sales are your best bet. If you feel comfortable using other online "sale" apps or websites like OfferUp or Facebook community "garage sale" groups then go for it.

o Play It Again Sports typically marks their stuff waaaay up.

o Avoid at all costs buying anything brand new, like from Dick's. After all, this is Building a Garage Gym on a Budget.

o Look for on-line or local clearance sales by well-known manufacturers like Rogue Fitness or Perform Better.

o Also lookout for clearance or "garage sale" events from local manufacturers trying to get rid of older product versions. I went to one hosted by a local place and ended up with 2 really nice olympic barbells, a few bumper plates, plyo boxes, a couple kettlebells, and a push sled (altogether about a $900 value) and I paid just over $200.

o When buying olympic plates or dumbbells, do NOT pay more than $0.50/lb.

o Power Racks will usually go from $75 to $250 used.

o Olympic Bars will typically go from $50 to $150 used.

o When buying used kettlebells do NOT pay more than $0.75-$1.00/lb

o To really find something good on Craigslist you must check constantly. I downloaded a free Craigslist app on my phone specifically for this purpose. And make sure you use multiple spellings of different words. For instance, dumbbells can be dumbells, dumbell, dumb bells, dumb bell, or can be referred to as a barbell. Kettlebells can be kettlebell, kettle bell, kettleball, kettleballs, kettle ball, or kettle balls. Search carefully, and use every word you can think off. Only search one word at a time. Sometimes you check and then 5 minutes later a great piece of equipment at a great price pops up, but you don't check until an hour later and by that time it's already gone. Increase your chances of finding something by checking often. You want to find the deals right? Well, spending some extra time on Craigslist for a couple weeks won't cost you a dime. In fact, it will probably end up saving you a lot of money. About a month before writing this, I bought a brand new, untouched set of dumbbell pairs from 15lb to 50lb with a rack valued at about $500 and paid $75. Sometimes people don't know what they have, or they do know what they have and they need it gone quickly. Don't be afraid to make an offer as well, but please don't low ball people, especially on low-priced items. Don't be a jerk.